Fit by Fart:
Toot Your Horn to Good Health

Fit by Fart:
Toot Your Horn to Good Health

**A handbook of good nutrition by
Hope Scott Paul, MS, RD**

ISBN 978-0-557-11446-7

Cover created by the author.

Beans, beans, the magical fruit
The more we eat, the more we toot
The more we toot, the better we feel
So eat your beans with every meal!
- Anonymous

Preface

Fad diets usually involve some kind of strange or crazy scheme, cutting out whole food groups, making you eat your foods in a certain order, and other asinine things. Fad diets don't work. If they did, they wouldn't come and go with the breeze. Everyone would follow them. We'd all look like models, and there would be world peace. That obviously hasn't happened yet. Gimmicks aren't any better, either. Think about this the next time you see an ad for a diet pill/detox shake machine/weight-loss wrist band – if there truly were a huge scientific discovery that could help people lose weight, wouldn't it be huge news? Obesity is one of the biggest public health issues in this century; obesity increases risk for heart disease, diabetes, cancer, high blood pressure, high cholesterol, stroke, arthritis and breathing problems. Wouldn't a successful weight-loss pill or gadget win the Nobel Prize?

While there are many things that can influence a person's weight (like genes or working in a setting where you don't move around much), scientific evidence shows that food choices and exercise are also major factors of a person's weight. Research has shown that the best way to be at a healthy weight is to make healthful food choices, eat moderate amounts, and exercise daily. Unfortunately, that's not easy to put into infomercial form. Although it's sold in various forms, there's no scientifically safe and sound "quick fix" or "magic bullet" that you can use to lose 20 pounds overnight. If you do lose that much weight that quickly, please call your doctor. I have no idea how much weight you'll lose after you read this book; I'm not guaranteeing anything, because it's totally up to you. We know from research how to lose weight and keep it off – but you need to apply it to your life in a way that you can keep up with for the rest of your life. The purpose of this book is to try to package the "tough love" message of how to be at a healthy weight in a fun and interesting way, in a way that you can associate with and can apply to yourself.

Enjoy!

Dietitian Hope

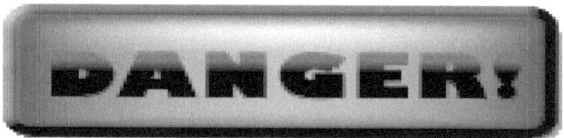

Do not skip ahead and look only for menu plans and recipes and read the last page. This book will self-destruct if you do not read the pages consecutively!

OK. The book is not really going to implode, but you will be missing out on the wit and intellect bursting forth from each page. That's a crime.

This book has not been funded nor approved by proctologists and gastroenterologists (butt and gut doctors), although I believe they would agree with all the material being presented.

Contents

Chapter 1

Fiber! What is it? Why do I need it?

Hope's Handy Hint: Need to have a good poop? Eat fiber. Remember that eating fiber is like Goldilocks and the Three Bears - not too much, or you'll be in trouble. Not too little, either. You need just the right amount. Moderation is central to most everything in life, including how to eat and especially in dealing with fiber. Fiber is amazing stuff – it can really help you to reach your weight goals, or it can really hurt you (sometimes quite literally!).

Fiber is stuff found in the plants we eat that your body cannot digest - it is sometimes known as "roughage" or "bulk." Since your body does not absorb it, fiber goes essentially unchanged from your stomach to your small intestine to your colon. There are two types of fiber. There's fiber that can break up in water (soluble) and fiber that cannot (insoluble). Soluble fiber turns into a sort of gel, which slows down how quickly food goes through your digestive system and helps your body to absorb important nutrients. Insoluble fiber does the opposite – it helps foods move more quickly through your stomach and intestines and adds bulk to your stool. In other words, it helps you poop.

Both kinds of fiber are important for a healthy digestive system and for preventing disease, but most people aren't concerned about how much fiber they eat. Fiber is being added to many packaged foods because most of us do not eat enough foods that are good sources of fiber. The focus is usually on fat, or carbs, or sugar, or something else. According to "What We Eat in America," part of the large National Health and Nutrition Examination Survey, most adults are getting about 15 grams of fiber per day.[1] That's about 50% of the recommended amount.

Eating the right amount of fiber each day may help you to:

- Lose weight, or stay at a healthy weight. Fiber-rich foods fill you up – you can actually feel fuller for fewer calories.

---

[1] Agricultural Research Service, U.S. Department of Agriculture. *Nutrient intakes from food: Mean amounts consumed per individual, one day, 2003-2004* [Data file]. Retrieved August 5, 2009 from http://www.ars.usda.gov/SP2UserFiles/Place/12355000/pdf/0304/Table_1_NIF.pdf .

- Lower your cholesterol levels. Gel-like soluble fiber may trap some cholesterol during digestion and keep it from going back into your blood stream (in other words, you poop out some cholesterol and that lowers your blood cholesterol levels).
- Have a healthy poop. In technical terms, fiber helps you to have a bulky, soft stool.
- Reduce your chances of getting: hemorrhoids (thanks to the healthy poop that won't make you strain); irritable bowel syndrome; and small pouches in your colon that may trap food particles (diverticular disease).

The motivation for this book and for talking so much about fiber is that **fiber** is the key, the missing ingredient in your weight loss and health goals. **In a nutshell, get the right amount of fiber you need each day from a variety of foods and you'll be at a healthy weight.** It's a little more complicated than that, but you get the gist. And it's not a good idea to eat snack or meal replacement bars with super amounts of fiber in them and to drink a fiber supplement drink. Variety is the spice of life – literally. If you eat just snack bars and supplement drinks with fiber, you miss out on all the food groups. Each food group provides you with many different vitamins, minerals, phytochemicals, antioxidants, and the things that haven't even been discovered yet. So to be healthy, you shouldn't eat the same few items throughout the day. Later you'll see how to get the right amount of fiber, calories, fat, and other important nutrients in a few easy steps (and on a budget, too!).

Hope's Handy Hint - The key to a lean, sexy, healthy body is to eat fruits and vegetables, whole grains, low fat dairy products, plant-based protein, a little lean meat, and some healthy fats – but all in moderation, along with a physically active lifestyle.

DIET MYTH-BUSTING

Before we go any further, we need to discuss and bust some prevalent and popular diet myths. Here are some common myths and the facts behind them:

1. MYTH: Sugar-free foods are calorie-free.

   Not necessarily. **While some sugar-free foods have almost no calories (like Crystal Light or sugar-free gum), other sugar-free foods can have the same amount of calories, or even more calories, than the regular version**. To make a sugar-free product tasty, fat is sometimes added. This additional fat can increase the amount of calories in the food. Be sure to compare the fat and calories in sugar-free and regular foods; make your decision based on this, as well as on the price of the product.

2. MYTH: Bread is bad – go low-carb.

   Bread, pasta, rice and other "high carb" foods are not evil. They can be good components of a healthful eating plan. These foods become high in fat in calories when they're loaded with butter, cheese, sugar and other high calorie foods. **Carbohydrates are an important source of fuel for your body, and not eating enough carbohydrates may be harmful for your health.** The minimum amount of carbohydrate you need each day is 130 grams. That's the amount in about 8 ½ slices of bread. Consuming fewer than 130 grams of carbohydrate a day may lead to ketosis, which is a buildup of ketones (partially broken-down fats) in your blood. Your body may produce high levels of uric acid because of these ketones, and this may lead to gout and kidney stones. Ketosis is *especially dangerous* for women who are pregnant and for people with diabetes or kidney disease. [2]

---

[2] Adapted from: Weight Information Network, National Institute of Diabetes and Digestive and Kidney Diseases, National Institutes of Health. (2009, March). *Weight loss and nutrition myths: How much do you really know?* [NIH Publication No. 04–4561]. Retrieved August 4, 2009 from http://win.niddk.nih.gov/publications/myths.htm.

3. MYTH: All the food you eat after 7:00 pm turns to fat.

    Your choice of food is more important than what time you're eating it. If you take in more calories than you need for the day, even from healthful foods, your body will store those extra calories. It doesn't matter if it's 3:00 in the afternoon or 3:00 in the morning – extra calories are extra calories. As you'll see in the sample menus, you can easily fit in an evening snack and lose weight, regardless of what time you have it. Your food choices need to fit into your overall healthful eating plan.[2]

4. MYTH: Certain foods burn fat.

    There are not any foods that burn/eat/destroy fat. If grapefruit or celery or cabbage could actually burn fat, no one would have any difficulty eating fruits and vegetables! **The only way to lose fat, and to lose weight, is to consume *slightly* fewer calories than your body requires.** Remember that you don't want to cut back on your calories too much, because you need a certain amount of calories to keep your body working properly and to be healthy. We'll go into more detail about this later .[2]

5. MYTH: You need to have a detox diet before you try to lose any weight.

    There is no standard "detox diet." That should be the first clue – standardization is key. **Our bodies are designed to remove efficiently and effectively most toxins we ingest via the kidneys and liver.** These toxins are then removed from your body when you go to the bathroom. There isn't any evidence that detox diets actually eliminate toxins from your body. Increased feelings of psychological well-being and feeling "lighter" or more focused may be due to the calorie restriction of detox diets. Talk with your doctor before going on a fast and/or a detox diet.[3]

---

[3] Adapted from: Mayo Foundation for Medical Education and Research. (2008). *Detox diets: Do they offer any health benefits?*. Retrieved September 2, 2009 from http://mayoclinic.com/health/detox-diets/AN01334.

6. MYTH: I need to use a colon cleanser.

A colon cleanser may be recommended before a procedure like a colonoscopy, but in general it isn't necessary and may even be harmful. **Your body is designed to eliminate waste and bacteria, so you don't need enemas or pills to do this.** There isn't much scientific evidence for or against colon cleansing, but it can increase your risk for dehydration and make your electrolytes (such as sodium, potassium, calcium, and bicarbonate) increase. This is a serious concern for people with kidney or heart disease. Always check with your primary doctor before you use a colon cleanser. If you're thinking about using a colon cleanser to relieve constipation, fiber control and healthful eating are better options. [4]

7. MYTH: The multivitamin I take everyday makes up for my poor eating habits.

No! A multivitamin is a dietary supplement, which means it is supposed to *SUPPLEMENT* what you have to eat, not to replace eating wholesome foods. **Whole foods are the best way to get vitamins and minerals.** Foods offer many benefits over supplements – foods are complex and contain many vitamins and minerals. Foods also offer dietary fiber and are more satisfying than swallowing a pill. Finally, foods have phytochemicals that may offer health benefits, as well as important things we haven't even discovered yet. [5]

8. MYTH: Water makes you lose weight.

Water may help you lose weight if you have it INSTEAD of a higher – calorie beverage, like soda pop, sweet tea, and alcohol. Water itself is not a magic bullet. You lose weight when you take in fewer calories than your body requires to

---

[4]Adapted from: Mayo Foundation for Medical Education and Research. (2008). *Colon cleansers: Do they really work?*. Retrieved September 2, 2009 from http://mayoclinic.com/health/colon-cleansing/AN00065.
[5] Adapted from: Mayo Foundation for Medical Education and Research. (2008). *Dietary supplements: Nutrition in a pill?*. Retrieved September 6, 2009 from http://www.mayoclinic.com/health/supplements/NU00198.

stay at your current weight. **By substituting water for a beverage with calories (like regular soda pop), you may take in fewer calories and thereby lose weight.**

9. MYTH: Sugar causes diabetes.

Sugar *does not* cause diabetes. **Sugar usually *does* increase the amount of calories in a given food. Over-eating these calorie-dense foods may cause you to gain weight, and obesity is a risk factor for diabetes.** Lack of exercise also plays a role in weight gain and increases a person's risk for diabetes. To sum it up, eating foods high in sugar may cause you to eat more calories than you need. Consuming extra calories leads to weight gain. Being overweight or obese puts you at increased risk for diabetes.[6]

10. MYTH: Weight loss pills and supplements are a good way to lose weight.

Weight-loss pills and herbal supplements that claim to be "natural" can be very dangerous. **These items are regulated only as a dietary supplement, not as a medication, and therefore don't have to prove if they're safe and effective.** These pills and supplements can have unidentified ingredients in them and can contain toxic levels of ingredients. Weight-loss pills and herbal supplements can also interact adversely with both prescription and non-prescription medications you may be taking. There are a few FDA-approved weight-loss medications available if you truly want to have a "weight loss pill," but this option should be discussed thoroughly with your doctor to see if it's an appropriate option for you.[2]

11. MYTH: I have to drink red wine for heart health.

Do **NOT** start drinking alcohol just to receive heart health benefits. **IF** you already drink and **AFTER** you have a long talk with your doctor, **MODERATE** alcohol consumption

---

[6] Adapted from: American Dietetic Association. (2008). *Nutrition myth: Sugar causes diabetes*. Retrieved September 1, 2009 from http://www.eatright.org/cps/rde/xchg/ada/hs.xsl/home_16467_ENU_HTML.htm.

may be beneficial to reducing your risk of heart disease. "Moderate" alcohol consumption means 1 drink per day for women, 2 drinks per day for men. 1 drink = 1- 12 oz beer, 4 oz of wine (most wine glasses are 10 oz), 1.5 oz of 80-proof liquor (a shot), or 1 oz of 100-proof liquor. There are many risks that go along with drinking more alcohol, such as alcoholism, high blood pressure, obesity, stroke, breast cancer, suicide, and accidents. **The American Heart Association does NOT recommend drinking wine or other alcohol to get health benefits; instead, it recommends reducing your risk of heart disease by lowering your blood pressure and cholesterol, being at a healthy weight, exercising daily, and eating a healthy diet.**[7]

---

[7] American Heart Association. (n.d.). *Alcohol, wine, and cardiovascular disease.* Retrieved September 28, 2009 from http://www.americanheart.org/presenter.jhtml?identifier=4422 .

Chapter 2

The more fiber you eat, the better?

Hope's Handy Hint: Please do not eat cardboard, or foods that seem like cardboard. There are many better options for increasing your fiber intake that are better-looking, tastier, and much more satisfying!

You may be thinking, "The more fiber I eat, the better?" **NO!** It's all about getting the right amount of fiber, fat, and fluid. Let me tell you a story about my mother. My mom is well-read on nutrition presented in the popular media. She was eating all the "superfoods" touted by the articles that come up when you check your email – she was eating flax seed, almonds, salmon, blueberries, cooking with olive oil, and so on. Because she was making an effort to read about healthful eating and to apply it to her own life, she was upset when routine blood work came back and the doctor said that her cholesterol was high. She asked her dietitian daughter to tell her why that happened, if she was eating "all the right things." When I asked her to tell me what she ate in a typical day and entered it into a handy-dandy nutrition analysis program, the problem was very obvious. Her calorie intake was OK, but half her calories were coming from fat and she was consuming only about 12 grams of fiber (which is actually the average intake for women in the U.S.). I found out my mom wasn't eating any bread, rice, any of those really "carb-y" foods. So our conversation went something like this:

Dietitian Hope: "Momma, you're not eating any fiber! Not much from the grains group."

Hope's Mom: "No, I don't really eat bread or anything like that. I don't want to eat too much."

Dietitian Hope: "But you need to eat more fiber! You need to eat some carbs. You want half of your calories to be from carbohydrate. They're not evil. And, compared to your calorie intake, you're eating too much fat."

And so my mother stocked up on double-fiber bread, high-fiber cereal, crackers with lots of fiber, and fiber-loaded granola bars (and

I'm sure much of it looked like cardboard). About 2 weeks later, following up on our previous conversation, she was even more upset:

Hope's Mom:	"I got all kinds of fiber stuff and have been eating it every day ... I've gained 5 pounds and I'm seriously bloated! What the heck?!?"
Dietitian Hope:	"OK. Tell me what you're having now and we'll see what's wrong."
Hope's Mom:	"Well, I have a cup of this super-fiber cereal for breakfast, a fiber granola bar for a snack with some fruit, a sandwich on double-fiber bread with some broccoli...."

With a little investigating and again turning to my handy nutrition analysis program, we discovered my mom was taking in 1,000 calories more per day than she had been and had jumped to having 40 grams of fiber per day. No wonder she was mad at me and extremely tootsie. She went from one end of the spectrum to another, certainly not something you should do.

How much fiber do you and my mom need to get every day?

If you are a:	Your daily fiber intake should be:
Man, age 14 - 50	38 grams
Man, age 50 and older	30 grams
Woman , age 9 -18	26 grams
Woman, age 19 – 50	25 grams
Woman, age 50 and older	21 grams
Woman, pregnant or breastfeeding	28-29 grams

Adapted from: Food and Nutrition Board, Institute of Medicine, National Academies. (2005). Table: Dietary Reference Intakes: Macronutrients. *Dietary Reference Intakes for Energy, Carbohydrate. Fiber, Fat, Fatty Acids, Cholesterol, Protein, and Amino Acids (2002/2005)*. Retrieved August 11, 2009 from http://www.iom.edu/Object.File/Master/7/300/Webtablemacro.pdf.

What do 38 grams of fiber look like in a day of eating, you ask? They could look something like this:

<u>Breakfast</u>:	a slice of whole wheat toast, 1 cup shredded wheat cereal, 1 medium peach, ½ cup blueberries (= 12 grams of fiber)
<u>Snack</u>:	16 cherries (= about 3 grams of fiber)
<u>Lunch</u>:	2 slices whole wheat bread (for a sandwich), ¾ cup cooked snow peas (= 9.5 grams of fiber)
<u>Snack</u>:	8 baby carrots, 7 reduced-fat Triscuits (= about 5 grams of fiber)
<u>Dinner</u>:	¾ cup cooked brown rice, ¾ cup cooked broccoli, ¾ cup cooked cauliflower (= about 10 grams of fiber)

Likewise, about 25 grams of fiber would look like a modified version of the above:

<u>Breakfast</u>:	a slice of whole wheat toast, ½ cup shredded wheat cereal, ½ of a medium peach, ½ cup blueberries (= 9 grams of fiber)
<u>Snack</u>:	16 cherries (= about 3 grams of fiber)
<u>Lunch</u>:	1 slice whole wheat bread (for ½ a sandwich), ½ cup cooked snow peas (= about 5 grams of fiber)
<u>Snack</u>:	6 baby carrots, 3 reduced-fat Triscuits (= about 3 grams of fiber)
<u>Dinner</u>:	½ cup cooked brown rice, ½ cup cooked broccoli, ½ cup cooked cauliflower (= about 6 grams of fiber)

You wouldn't eat just these foods, of course. The suggestions listed are just the fiber-containing foods. In chapter 7 you'll see all the food you need in a day of healthful eating, not just the foods with fiber.

As we all know, calories are important to stay at a healthy weight and to remain healthy. Weight loss and weight gain are actually quite simple – it's all about balance. Think of it like a see-saw. To balance a see-saw, each side has to be equally weighted. One side (the calories you eat each day) has to be very similar to the other side (how many calories you need each day). If you eat more calories than your body needs, your body will store those calories, the see-saw will tip to one side, and you'll gain weight. If you eat fewer calories than your body needs, your body will need to make up the difference between how many calories you're eating and how many calories you need by utilizing some of your stored energy (a.k.a. "weight"). This will tip the see-saw the other way, and you'll lose weight. Remember, though, that your body requires a certain amount of calories for basic functions, like making your heart beat, churning up the food in your stomach, fueling the muscles in your legs so you can walk, and so on. Going back to our example of the see-saw, abandoning one side of the see-saw (in other words, not eating much, or eating very little) throws everything off balance. If the see-saw in your life is way off balance, there are many wonderful healthcare professionals who can help you get everything back on track. Later we'll talk about how to cut back on your calories SLIGHTLY so you keep your body healthy and lose weight in a slow, healthy way.

So how many calories do you require each day for your body to be healthy and to function properly? Most men need approximately 2000- 3000 calories per day, while most women need 1600 – 2400 calories per day. You can find the specific amount of daily calories you need for your gender, age, and daily exercise level in the following charts:

	Men		
Age	**<30 minutes exercise per day* (Sedentary)**	**30 – 60 minutes of exercise per day* (Moderately Active)**	**>60 minutes of exercise per day* (Active)**
19-20	2600	2800	3000
21-25	2400	2800	3000
26-30	2400	2600	3000
31-35	2400	2600	3000
36-40	2400	2600	2800
41-45	2200	2600	2800
46-50	2200	2400	2800
51-55	2200	2400	2800
56-60	2200	2400	2600
61-65	2000	2400	2600
66-70	2000	2200	2600
71-75	2000	2200	2600
76 and older	2000	2200	2400

Adapted from: U.S. Department of Agriculture, Center for Nutrition Policy and Promotion. (April 2005). *MyPyramid food intake pattern calorie levels.* Retrieved August 27, 2009 From http://www.mypyramid.gov/downloads/MyPyramid_Calorie_Levels.pdf.

*in ADDITION to usual daily activities

Age	Women		
	<30 minutes exercise per day* (Sedentary)	30 – 60 minutes of exercise per day* (Moderately Active)	>60 minutes of exercise per day* (Active)
19-20	2000	2200	2400
21-25	2000	2200	2400
26-30	1800	2000	2400
31-35	1800	2000	2200
36-40	1800	2000	2200
41-45	1800	2000	2200
46-50	1800	2000	2200
51-55	1600	1800	2200
56-60	1600	1800	2200
61-65	1600	1800	2000
66-70	1600	1800	2000
71-75	1600	1800	2000
76 and older	1600	1800	2000

Adapted from: U.S. Department of Agriculture, Center for Nutrition Policy and Promotion. (April 2005).
MyPyramid food intake pattern calorie levels. Retrieved August 27, 2009
From http://www.mypyramid.gov/downloads/MyPyramid_Calorie_Levels.pdf

*in ADDITION to usual daily activities

And now... fat! Fat is not evil. We need to have fat in our diet. Fat provides a lot of good things for your body, like fat-soluble vitamins (vitamins A, D, E & K), cushioning and insulation for your organs, and energy. The 2005 *Dietary Guidelines for Americans* recommends that fat should make up 20 to 35 percent of all your calories, if you're age 19 or older. Kids (age 4 and older) and teenagers should aim for 25 to 35 percent, while kids age 2 to 3 need 30 to 35 percent.[8] Too much fat (more than 35 percent) may affect your cholesterol and triglyceride levels, and increase your risk of heart disease. On the other hand, too little fat (less than 20 percent) increases your risk of not getting enough vitamin E and essential fatty acids.

---

[8] U.S. Department of Health and Human Services and U.S. Department of Agriculture. (2005). Chapter 6: Fats. *Dietary Guidelines for Americans, 2005* (6th ed.). Washington, D.C.: U.S. Government Printing Office. Retrieved August 10, 2009 from http://www.health.gov/dietaryguidelines/dga2005/document/html/chapter6.htm.

Omega-3 and omega-6 fatty acids are considered to be the essential fatty acids. Our bodies can make all the fatty acids we need except for these two, so we have to get omega-3 and omega-6 fatty acids from our foods. Omega-3 and Omega-6 fatty acids are part of the structure of cell membranes. They also are precursors to eicosanoids, which help regulate blood pressure, blood clotting, and the body's immune response to injury and infection, among other things. You can see how many grams of fat you need each day, based on your calorie level and the percent of your calories you are getting from fat, in the following chart:

Calorie Level	20% Calories from Fat	25% Calories from Fat	30% Calories from Fat
1600	36 grams	44 grams	53 grams
1800	40 grams	50 grams	60 grams
2000	44 grams	56 grams	67 grams
2200	49 grams	61 grams	73 grams
2400	53 grams	67 grams	80 grams

These numbers for fat grams probably don't make any sense to you right now. To give you an idea of what they mean in real world eating, look at the sample menus in chapter 7. These menus have approximately 25 - 30 percent of their calories from fat. The suggested foods listed in the menus should give you an idea of how to get the right amount of fat.

In addition to the right amount, it is equally important to get the right kinds of fats – most of the fat you eat should be from the "better" fats, monounsaturated and polyunsaturated fats. You want to limit how much saturated and *trans* fat you eat (otherwise known as the "bad" fats). The American Heart Association recommends the saturated fat you eat should be less than 7 percent of your total calories (in other words, don't eat much saturated fat) and the *trans* fat you eat should be less than 1 percent of all your calories (in other words, avoid *trans* fat).

So what in the world are these fats and what foods are they in? Saturated fat is found primarily in animal products (like whole milk, regular cheese, bacon, etc.) and some plant oils, while *trans* fats are found in many fried foods, baked goods, and snack foods. Each type of fat has an effect on heart health, as you see here:

Type of Fat:	Food Sources:	Effect on Heart Health:
Saturated	• Mainly from animals: beef, lamb, pork, poultry with skin, beef fat, lard, cream, butter, cheese, and other whole and reduced-fat dairy products. • Some from plants: palm, palm kernel, and coconut oils.	• Raise bad cholesterol level • Foods high in saturated fats may also be high in cholesterol • Increase risk of heart disease
Trans	• Baked goods – pastries, biscuits, muffins, cakes, pie crusts, doughnuts, cookies • Fried foods – French fries, fried chicken, breaded chicken nuggets and breaded fish • Snack foods – popcorn, crackers • Traditional stick margarine and vegetable shortening	• Raise bad cholesterol • May lower good cholesterol • Increase risk of heart disease
Monounsaturated	• Vegetable oils- olive, canola, peanut, and sesame • Avocados, many nuts and seeds	• Reduce bad cholesterol • May lower risk of heart disease
Polyunsaturated	• Vegetable oils – soybean, corn, safflower and sunflower • Fatty fish – salmon, tuna, mackerel, herring, and trout • Most nuts and seeds	• Reduce bad cholesterol • May lower risk of heart disease

Adapted from: American Heart Association. (2008). *Meet the Fats: Some are bad, some are better.* Retrieved August 19, 2009 from http://www.americanheart.org/downloadable/heart/1210953558714Large%20Print%20Pocket%20Guide%20PDF%20for%20Web.pdf.

Since the "better" fats are good for your heart health, can you eat as much of them as you want? **No!** All fats, whether they're from bacon fat or olive oil, have about the same amount of calories. The key is to eat monounsaturated and polyunsaturated fats **INSTEAD** of saturated and *trans* fat, not to add the "better" fats to what you're already eating. Like we already discussed, eating extra calories, or more calories than your body needs, may lead to weight gain even if those calories are from healthful foods.

So how do you know how much fat and how many calories a food has, or what kind of fat it is, or how much fiber is in the food? By looking at the Nutrition Facts label on the package! An essential step to being an informed consumer is to look at the Nutrition Facts label on packaged foods to see what's really in the food. Where do we start with the Nutrition Facts label?

- **Serving Size** – this is a standardized amount determined by the government, useful in helping you to compare the calories and nutrients (protein, carbs, fat, etc.) of similar products.
- **Servings Per Container** – all the information listed on the Nutrition Facts panel goes along with the Serving Size listed at the top. If the serving size is 1 cup and you eat 2 cups, you have to double all the nutrition information listed.
- **Fat and Cholesterol** – remember that you want to limit your intake of saturated and trans fats, get most of your fat from the "better" mono and polyunsaturated fats, and get the right amount of total fat. Try not to consume more than 300 milligrams of cholesterol per day (less than 200 milligrams per day for some people with heart health issues).
- **Fiber** – you already know how important fiber is. A food is considered to be a good source of fiber if it has 3 grams or more per serving, and an excellent source if it has 5 grams or more per serving.
- **Nutrients** – vitamin A, vitamin C, calcium, and iron are important nutrients for overall health. Choose foods with higher amounts of these nutrients.

Let's take a look at a Nutrition Facts label:

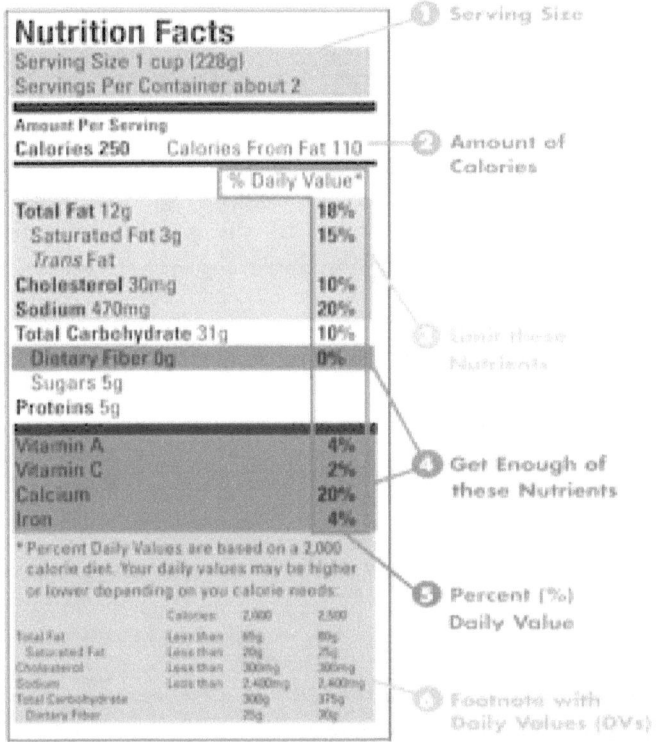

Source: U.S. Food and Drug Administration. (2006, October). *A key to choosing healthful foods: Using the nutrition facts on the food label.* Retrieved August 19, 2009 from http://www.fda.gov/Food/ResourcesForYou/Consumers/ucm079449.htm.

> **Hope's Handy Hint** - For the "Get Enough of these Nutrients" section, use the % Daily Value as a guide. 5% of the Daily Value or less is considered to be low, 10 - 19% is considered to be a "good source," and 20% or more is considered to be high or an "excellent source" or "rich in" that nutrient.

Now that you know how to find out what the serving size of a food is, how can you tell if what you're eating is a serving? Compare your portion size (the amount you *choose* to have) to objects that are similar in size to the serving size of the food (the **standardized amount** listed on the nutrition facts label). For example:

A fist = about 1 cup

A cupcake wrapper = ½ cup of cooked rice or pasta, or hot or cold cereal

Palm of your hand = 3 ounces of lean meat

A deck of cards = 3 ounces of lean meat

Tip of your thumb = 1 teaspoon

Tip of your index finger = ½ teaspoon

Thumb, from tip to 2nd joint = 1 ounce of low fat cheese

4 dice = 1 ounce of low fat cheese

A Handful = 1 – 2 ounces of snack food

A ping-pong ball = 2 tablespoons

3 thumb tips = 1 tablespoon

A baseball = 1 medium fruit

½ a baseball = ½ cup fresh, frozen, or canned fruits or vegetables

Remember that everyone's hand size is different, so these comparisons are just a guide. The best way to be sure about your portion sizes is to use kitchen measuring cups and measuring spoons and a food scale.

There are a lot of buzz words on food packages that can be helpful, confusing, or a little of both. Phrases like "**low-fat**," "**low sodium**," "**sugar-free**" and "**natural**" are usually on the front of a food package and are very noticeable. Do you know what these nutrient claims (as the phrases are called) really mean when you see them on a food package? Here is a general guide to the nutrient claims and their definitions:

Low Calorie	40 calories or less per serving
Low Fat	3 grams or less of fat per serving
Low Sodium	140 mg or less of sodium per serving
Reduced	25% less per serving than comparison food
Light or Lite	33.3% fewer calories or 50% less fat per serving than comparison food
Lean	Less than 10 grams of fat, 4.5 grams of saturated fat, and 95 milligrams of cholesterol per serving
Extra Lean	Less than 5 grams of fat, 2 grams of saturated fat and 95 milligrams of cholesterol per serving

Source: American Dietetic Association & American Diabetes Association. (2005). Table 3: Nutrient claims on food labels. The diabetes carbohydrate & fat gram guide (3rd ed.).

The terms "Natural" and "Organic" are also found with some regularity on food packages. Most people aren't aware of the true definitions of these terms:

- **"Natural,"** according to the U.S. Food & Drug Administration, means foods that are minimally processed and free of synthetic preservatives; artificial sweeteners, colors, flavors and other artificial additives; growth hormones; antibiotics; hydrogenated oils; stabilizers; and emulsifiers.[9] **This term applies broadly to foods, and most "natural" foods are not subject to any more government controls than are other foods.**

- The U.S. Department of Agriculture has specific guidelines for organic foods. **"Organic" food differs from conventionally produced food in the way it is grown, handled, and processed, but it doesn't necessarily mean the food is safer or more healthful.** Organic crops are raised without using most conventional pesticides, petroleum-based fertilizers, or manure (otherwise known as feces) based fertilizers. Animals raised on an organic operation must be fed organic feed and given access to the outdoors. The animals are not given antibiotics or growth hormones; genetic engineering, ionizing radiation, and feces are prohibited in organic production and

---

[9] Food Marketing Institute. (n.d.).Natural and organic foods. *FMI Backgrounder*. Retrieved August 24, 2009 from http://www.fda.gov/ohrms/dockets/dockets/06p0094/06p-0094-cp00001-05-Tab-04-Food-Marketing-Institute-vol1.pdf .

handling. Natural (non-synthetic) substances are allowed, while synthetic substances are prohibited.[10] **In short, organic is better for the environment**.

Here's an example to help you see the difference between "natural" and "organic." "Natural" peanut butter may list peanuts as the only ingredient. However, those peanuts may have been grown using pesticides, petroleum-based fertilizers, or manure-based fertilizers, and the seeds used to grow the peanuts may have been genetically modified. Ergo, my "natural" peanut butter may not have been made in an Earth-friendly way. It can be hard to decide between "natural" and "organic" foods. The best option, however, is to eat locally and sustainably grown foods, or to grow or raise your own foods in an environmentally sound way.

Finally, onto the fluid. According to the Institute of Medicine, drinking when you're thirsty and drinking beverages with meals are enough to stay hydrated. The Institute of Medicine has established an AI (short for adequate intake) for water. The AI is defined as the amount that will probably meet the needs for almost everyone in a healthy population. Water can come from beverages (like drinking water, juice, tea, coffee, and soda) as well as from moisture in foods (like watermelon, soup, cucumbers, moist meats, etc.).[11] Although you can confirm how much fluid you need each day with your own registered dietitian, the general recommendations for water from beverages are:

Men (age 19 and older)	12 ½ cups
Women (age 19 and older)	About 9 cups
Pregnant Women	10 cups
Breastfeeding Women	13 cups

Source: Food and Nutrition Board, Institute of Medicine, National Academies. (2004). Table: *Dietary Reference Intakes: Water, potassium, sodium, chloride, and sulfate*. Retrieved August 19, 2009 from http://www.iom.edu/Object.File/Master/20/004/0.pdf

---

[10] National Organic Program, U.S. Department of Agriculture. (2008, April). *Background information*. Retrieved August 24, 2009 from
http://www.ams.usda.gov/AMSv1.0/getfile?dDocName=STELDEV3004443&acct=nopgeninfo.
[11] Food and Nutrition Board, Institute of Medicine, National Academies. (2004). Table: Dietary Reference Intakes: Electrolytes and water. Taken from *Dietary Reference Intakes: Water, potassium, sodium, chloride, and sulfate*. Retrieved August 19, 2009 from http://www.iom.edu/Object.File/Master/20/004/0.pdf

Remember that this isn't strictly cups of water – everything you drink counts toward your water intake, but some beverages are better than others. In Chapter 5 you'll learn about liquid calories and the best beverages for your body and for your bank account.

Chapter 3

How do I eat the right amount of fiber??

The first step is to slightly modify how you are already eating. Sounds simple, right? It is. A good first step is to have whole wheat or whole grain bread instead of white bread. Use your food label-reading skills to choose breads with 3 grams of fiber per serving. If you can't switch completely, try using "white wheat" bread for a short while and then transition to whole wheat bread. Switching to whole grain products and eating more fruit and vegetables can help you boost how much fiber you get each day. Try to include more fiber-rich foods into your everyday eating. In general, whole grains, beans, fruits, and vegetables are good ways to get fiber. The following table has examples of other easy switches you can make to get more fiber:

The switch to make:	You'll boost your fiber intake by:
1 slice whole wheat bread instead of white bread	3 grams
1 cup of brown rice instead of white rice	3 grams
1 cup of whole wheat spaghetti instead of white spaghetti	4 grams
1 cup of plain Cheerios instead of Rice Krispies or Special K	3 grams
1 whole orange instead of 4 ounces of orange juice	3 grams
A medium baked potato with the skin instead of 1 cup instant mashed potatoes	2.5 grams
1 cup of kidney beans for some of the ground beef in chili or meatloaf	13 grams

Source: USDA National Nutrient Database for Standard Reference. Retrieved August 18, 2009 from http://www.nal.usda.gov/fnic/foodcomp/search/index.html

Hope's Handy Hint: Try adding no-salt-added canned black beans to many of your savory or meat-based dishes for additional fiber and some extra- lean protein.

Since everyone loves lists in a diet book, here is a list with a sampling of foods and their fiber content:

Food	Amount	Fiber Content
Navy Beans (cooked)	1 cup	19 grams
Lentils (cooked)	1 cup	15.6 grams
Black beans (cooked)	1 cup	15 grams
Kidney beans (cooked)	1 cup	13.8 grams
Chickpeas (cooked)	1 cup	12.5 grams
Baked Beans	1 cup	10.5 grams
Artichokes (cooked)	1 medium	10 grams
Peas (cooked from frozen)	1 cup	8.8 grams
Mixed vegetables (cooked from frozen)	1 cup	8 grams
Raspberries (raw)	1 cup	8 grams
Blackberries (raw)	1 cup	7.6 grams
Spaghetti/marinara sauce	1 cup	6.5 grams
Chopped Broccoli (cooked from frozen)	1 cup	5.5 grams
Collards (cooked)	1 cup	5.3 grams
Pear (raw)	1 medium	5 grams
Baked sweet potato, with skin	1 medium	4.8 grams
Carrots (cooked from frozen)	1 cup	4.8 grams
Baked white potato, with skin	1 medium	4.6 grams
Sweet corn (canned)	1 cup	4.2 grams
Oatmeal	1 cup	4 grams
Almonds	1 oz (24 nuts)	3.5 grams
Brown rice	1 cup	3.5 grams
Strawberries (raw)	1 cup	3.3 grams
Orange (raw)	1 medium	3.1 grams
Banana	1 medium	3.1 grams
Applesauce	1 cup	3.1 grams

Wild Rice	1 cup	3 grams
Cabbage (cooked)	1 cup	2.9 grams
Mixed nuts (dry roasted)	1 oz	2.6 grams

Source: USDA National Nutrient Database for Standard Reference, Release 20; Fiber, total dietary (g) content of selected foods per common measure, sorted by nutrient content. Retrieved August 18, 2009 from http://www.nal.usda.gov/fnic/foodcomp/Data/SR20/nutrlist/sr20w291.pdf

Just like making substitutions to increase your fiber intake, small changes can help you to cut back on how much fat you eat as well.

The switch to make:	You'll cut your fat intake by:
1 cup of skim milk instead of whole milk	8 grams
1 cup evaporated skim milk instead of heavy cream in a recipe	87.5 grams
½ cup low fat (1%) cottage cheese instead of regular (4%) cottage cheese	4 grams
2 tablespoons of Fat-free sour cream or fat free plain yogurt instead of regular sour cream	4.5 grams
2 egg whites instead of 1 whole egg	5 grams
2 tablespoons of Low-fat cream cheese instead of regular cream cheese	5.5 grams
2 teaspoons of whipped butter instead of stick butter	3.5 grams
2 tablespoons of light balsamic vinaigrette instead of Ranch dressing	13 grams
1 ounce turkey bacon instead of regular bacon	7.5 grams
½ cup Applesauce in place of ½ c oil in baked goods	109 grams
Non-stick cooking spray instead of a pat of butter (to prevent sticking)	4 grams
3 oz 90% lean ground beef instead of regular (75%) ground beef	5.5 grams
1 tablespoon light mayo instead of regular mayo	7 grams

Source: USDA National Nutrient Database for Standard Reference, Release 20. Retrieved August 18, 2009 from http://www.nal.usda.gov/fnic/foodcomp/search/index.html

Divided Plate

A great way to get a balanced meal and the right portion sizes is to use the "Divided Plate" method to serve meals for yourself and for your family. Start with drawing an imaginary line down the middle of your dinner plate (a 9-inch plate is a good size):

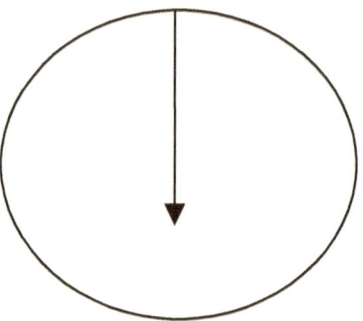

Now, fill half your plate with **non-starchy vegetables**, such as broccoli, carrots, salad greens, zucchini, or green beans.

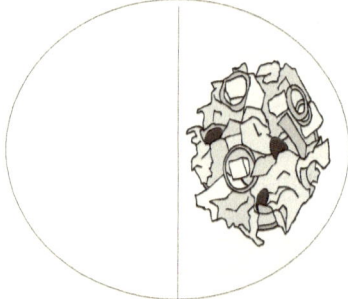

Divide the empty side of your plate in half, so you have two quarters.

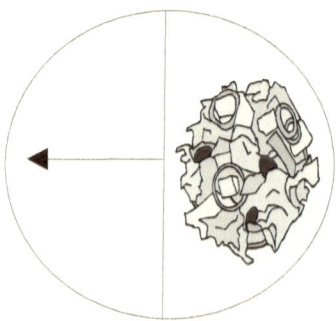

Fill one quarter up with **starchy foods** – either starchy vegetables like corn, peas, and potatoes, or with a grain, like brown rice, whole wheat spaghetti, or a whole wheat dinner roll. **If your portion is bigger than the allotted quarter of your plate, your portion size is too big.**

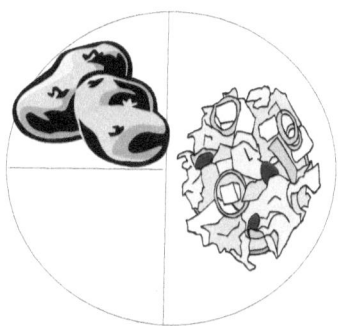

Fill the last quarter of your plate with protein foods. Put protein such as lean beef or pork (with the visible fat trimmed off), chicken (without the skin), fish (not breaded, but a plain fillet), an egg, beans, or tofu in this portion of your plate. The same portioning rule applies with protein foods - **if your portion is bigger than the allotted ¼ of your plate, you're having too much**.

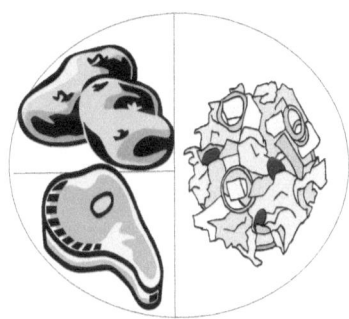

Round out your meal with a glass of skim or 1% milk and a small dish of fruit. You've got a great balanced lunch or dinner meal!

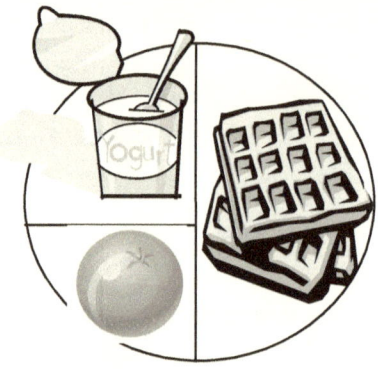

For breakfast meals, use the same strategy of having a half plate and two quarters. This time, fill half your plate with starchy food, such as whole wheat pancakes, whole grain cereal, whole wheat toast, or whole grain waffles. Put a protein food in one of the quarters – an egg, low fat yogurt, or low-fat cottage cheese. Put fruit in the other quarter. Another delicious, balanced meal!

Chapter 4

I don't want to have digestive distress!

<u>Hope's Handy Hint</u> - **Everybody poops. Everybody has gas**. In fact, you should see your doctor if you are *NOT* **pooping** and *NOT* **having gas**. You want to avoid fecal impaction, which is exactly what it sounds like: a large mass of dry, hard stool in the rectum, which may be so hard it can't come out of the body. Gross. Diarrhea isn't good, either. Diarrhea may be caused by many different things. Definitely see your doctor if you have chronic diarrhea, or diarrhea that lasts for more than 3 days. A "normal" bowel movement may be different for everyone, so go by what's normal for you.

During a summer vacation with my family I spent a good part of breakfast one morning talking up oatmeal to my then 4-year-old niece. It was one of my favorite conversations about the benefits of a fiber-rich food and bowel movements.

Aunt Dietitian Hope:	"Mmm! I LOVE oatmeal! It's my favorite breakfast food."
Dietitian Hope's niece:	"It looks funny and it's gloopy."
Aunt Dietitian Hope:	"Oh, but it's yummy and so good for me!"
Dietitian Hope's niece:	"Why is it good for you?" (eyeing the oatmeal speculatively)
Aunt Dietitian Hope:	"Well, it makes my tummy feel nice after I've been asleep all night because it's nice and warm. It helps me keep from getting too hungry when I'm playing before lunch. And it helps me to go to the bathroom."
Dietitian Hope's niece:	(eyes widening) "Will it help me poop?"
Aunt Dietitian Hope:	"Yep."
Dietitian Hope's niece:	(eyes even bigger, but now whispering) "Will it help me poop soft?"
Aunt Dietitian Hope:	"I bet it could definitely help."

That was all the convincing she needed to eat her bowl of oatmeal, so she dove right in. We enjoyed oatmeal together for breakfast through the whole vacation!

Few of us are as enthusiastic as my niece was to change bathroom habits, so remember to make changes SLOWLY. This will really help minimize digestive distress. Make just one change at a time, like the next chart demonstrates, especially if you haven't been eating many foods with fiber. As a young bride and a fresh-out-of-college dietitian I almost killed (or at least greatly distressed) my new husband with my overly-ambitious nutrition-enthusiast ways. My mother-in-law is an excellent down-home kind of cook, so my husband was raised with three big, hot meals a day. After our wedding, I stocked our new home with lots of fruits and veggies and whole grains. We had a nice high-fiber cereal and fruit for breakfast, a sandwich on whole-grain bread with lots of veggies for lunch, and some lean meat, veggies, and a whole grain for dinner. I cooked everything with non-stick cooking spray (no grease or lard to coat the pan) and sandwiches were always dry. He humored me for about 2 weeks with this way of eating, until one day he put down his fork and said he couldn't do it anymore (the way of eating, of course, not the marriage). He then admitted to me he'd been having "digestive distress" since the wedding and that he needed "non-binding food." In other words, he needed more fat and less fiber to help things move through his system. We were able to compromise by having some non-high fiber cereal, buttering toast and noodles, and eating fewer beans. A few weeks later we had both adjusted to my original eating plan – it just needed some transition time!

The moral of the story is do not jump into eating whole-grain, high-fiber everything. That's what my mom and my husband did (my husband less willingly than my mom), and both had unpleasant results. Take a few weeks and gradually introduce higher fiber foods into your diet. Depending on where you're at on the fiber intake scale, you'll want to take a few weeks to make small changes and to increase your fiber intake gradually. Try one change a week – see how that goes, let your body adjust to more fiber, and then make the next change. Make a schedule or a plan for yourself of what you're going to do. For example:

Week 1	Have a medium orange instead of orange juice with breakfast. Have white-wheat toast instead of white toast. Have an additional glass of water at work.
Week 2	Week 1 changes, plus brown rice instead of white rice for dinner. Add another glass of water.
Week 3	Week 1 &2 changes, plus broccoli with dinner.
Week 4	Week 1 – 3 changes, plus whole grain crackers instead of pretzels as a snack. Add a glass of water.
Week 5	Week 1-4 changes, plus low fat microwave popcorn as an evening snack instead of cookies.

Hope's Handy Hint - Make small changes. That's the easiest and the best thing to do. You don't have to change everything at once – in fact, that is usually a terrible idea. You make all these changes, you're really enthusiastic for a little while, and then you give up because it's too overwhelming. You're back to square one, or maybe even worse off. Just make a small change, something you can stick with, and build up from there. Small changes can really add up! And please don't think about this as a diet – a diet is something you do for a short period of time, in order to lose weight. Forget about that. Instead, make it your goal to be healthy and to take care of your body. If you make an effort to take care of your body for the long-term, your body is more likely to take care of you. Just think about it. If each of us does what we can to stay healthy we might be able to reduce medical costs, researchers could then focus on *preventing* disease (instead of working on *treating* disease), and we might get world peace after all!

Fart, toot, gas, flatulence, wind, cheese, crack splitters, butt burners ...

What's in a name? That which we call a fart
By any other name would smell as pungent.

What is a fart? Why does it smell? Everyone has thought about this at some point, because everyone has gas. Most people make 1 to 4 pints (2 to 8 cups) of intestinal gas each day, and the average person farts 14 to 23 times per day. Gas is mostly a combination of carbon dioxide, oxygen, nitrogen, hydrogen and sometimes methane. These gases are odorless – methane is not the culprit in the smelliness of a fart! The odor actually comes from sulfur, which is released by bacteria in the large intestine.

Your large intestine (or colon) naturally has harmless bacteria that break down the foods traveling through your gut. These bacteria are an essential part of digestion. As a by-product of breaking down the food for you, these bacteria produce gases. This is actually your fart! You're not the one making the gas, really – it's those little creatures in your colon. You're responsible for evacuating that gas. Sugars, starches, and fiber are digested in your large intestine (most other foods are digested in the small intestine), so they're the main foods responsible for gas. The sugars that cause gas are raffinose (a complex sugar found in beans as well as broccoli, brussel sprouts, and other veggies), lactose (the natural sugar in milk), fructose (naturally in onions, artichokes, pears, and wheat, and used to sweeten some soft drinks), and sorbitol (naturally found in fruits, and used as an artificial sweetener in many diet foods and sugar-free gums). Potatoes, corn, pasta, and wheat are starches that produce gas. And let's not forget about fiber - you should know all about fiber at this point. Remember that there are 2 types of fiber – insoluble and soluble. Insoluble passes through your gut without really changing, so it doesn't make much gas. Soluble, that gel-like fiber, is broken down by bacteria in the large intestine and definitely causes gas.

Gas is good and is a normal bodily function. Embrace it! Don't be embarrassed that you eat healthfully and have productive bacteria in residence.

Adapted from: National Digestive Diseases Information Clearinghouse, National Institute of Diabetes and Digestive and Kidney Diseases, National Institutes of Health. (2008, January). Gas in the digestive tract [NIH Publication No. 08–883]. Retrieved October 14, 2009 from http://digestive.niddk.nih.gov/ddiseases/pubs/gas/.

Chapter 5

I can't afford to buy "diet food" and feed other people too!

You don't have to buy "diet food." In fact, you shouldn't. You should purchase healthful choices for yourself and for your family. Healthful eating can actually help you to spend less on your groceries. Don't buy separate foods for yourself and for your kids. Your kids don't need salty snacks, candy, and soda pop, and neither do you. Just don't buy it. Snack foods, cookies, and sugary drinks can be expensive! Think about how much money you can save if you cut back on those extras. Plus, you might not be as tempted to have those items if they're not in the house. Don't get sucked into all the packaged foods designed for "dieting," either.

<u>**Hope's Handy Hint**</u>: If you really want to have a snack food, make your own 100 (some)-calorie packs. Get snack size food storage bags and your favorite snack food (pretzels, chips, etc.). Use your label-reading skills to see what a serving size is of that food, and measure it out into the baggie. Fill up the little baggies until you've emptied the big back of snack food. Now you have perfect portions! You won't overeat by eating straight out of the bag, you can get that snack fix in a modest way, and your snacks will last longer (since you won't be eating as much at one time).

The key to sticking to a budget and to eating healthful choices is having a plan! And plan some more! And stick with your plan! Think about ideas for what you are going to have for meals and snacks for the week. After you develop a general plan for meals, decide on a plan of attack. Grocery store circulars can become your best friend. Strategize and substitute to get the best bang for your buck. Base your menu plan around healthful items that may be on sale – for example, if chicken breast is on sale, have some chicken-based meals. If black beans are on sale, use black beans in tacos instead of ground beef. If you have storage space, stock up on these healthful items when they're on sale so you can always make a good, quick meal or snack:

- Instant brown rice
- Low-sodium canned chickpeas, black beans, kidney beans, etc
- Frozen and/or canned tuna and salmon
- Whole grain bread, English muffins, mini bagels
- Liquid egg substitute/
- Powdered egg whites
- Olive oil
- Vinegar (white wine, cider, red wine)
- Non-stick cooking spray
- Fat-free evaporated milk
- Natural peanut butter (the kind you have to stir)
- Low-sodium canned soup
- Tomato sauce
- Whole wheat spaghetti
- Oatmeal
- Low-fat yogurt and cottage cheese
- Frozen fruit or canned fruit in juice or water
- Frozen vegetables or no-salt-added canned vegetables

Fresh fruits and vegetables are your best option. Canned vegetables are usually high in sodium (or salt), and canned fruit that's packed in syrup has a lot of added sugar. However, using canned or frozen fruits and veggies is better than not having any. Try to get canned veggies that say "no salt added" and fruit that's packed in water or in juice, instead of in syrup. Canned and frozen foods can be a great way to eat healthfully on a budget. Frozen foods are especially handy when cooking for just 1 or 2 people. Be sure to look beyond the grocery store, too. If you live in an area with farmers' markets, check them out! Farmers' markets are an excellent way to get great produce at a good price and to support local agriculture. Many farmers' markets accept both WIC and seniors' vouchers for produce.

Hope's Handy Hint: Number 2 produce, the produce that's not as pretty or might be banged up a little, usually comes in large quantities for a little price. Most vegetables (and fruits, too) can be frozen very easily. Wash the vegetables thoroughly and cut them up into usable sizes (like slices), lay them out on a cookie sheet, and stick the cookie sheet in your freezer. Leave the sheet there for a few hours, take the sheet out of the freezer once everything's really hard, and then put the frozen vegetable slices into freezer bags. Now you can enjoy those veggies throughout the year! Fruits like peaches, strawberries, and blueberries can be frozen in the same way as well. If you're old school (or en vogue, depending on your perspective), canning is another option. Tomatoes can be cold-packed in water pretty easily, and cold-packed bell peppers in a vinegar and water mixture are tasty, too.

Remember the Liquid Calories

Calories aren't found only in food, but in beverages as well. The liquid calories you have should be nutrient-dense, which means that they should have lots of vitamins and minerals. What you put in coffee and tea adds up, and some "coffee" drinks at coffee and donut shops are loaded with unnecessary sugar and fat. Soda pop, energy drinks, fruit-ades, fruit punch, sweet tea and lemonade all can add lots of unwelcome calories (and don't give you vitamins and minerals like other healthful beverages do).

The best, least-expensive options for the whole family:

1. **Water.**

2. **Fat-Free (skim) milk** or **1% milk.** (Children age 2 and older should be drinking 1% or skim milk[12], but follow your pediatrician's recommendation for your child.)

3. **100% fruit juice.** (Children age 1 to 6 should limit fruit juice to 4 to 6 ounces per day, or ½ cup; children age 7 to 18 should limit fruit juice to 8 to 12 ounces per day, or 1 to 1 ½ cups[13]. Adults should also go easy on the fruit juice – remember that 4 ounces of fruit juice is about 60 calories, and that fruit juice counts toward your total amount of fruit for the day.)

---

[12] U.S. Department of Health & Human Services. (2005). Chapter 12: Healthier children. In *A healthier you: Based on the 2005 Dietary Guidelines for Americans*. Retrieved August 11, 2009 from http://www.health.gov/dietaryguidelines/dga2005/healthieryou/html/chapter12.html.
[13] American Academy of Pediatrics, Committee on Nutrition. (2001, May). The use and misuse of fruit juice in pediatrics. *Pediatrics, 107*, 5, p. 1210 – 1213. Retrieved August 12, 2009 from http://aappolicy.aappublications.org/cgi/reprint/pediatrics;107/5/1210.pdf.

Hope's Handy Hint: If you're a soda pop drinker, use seltzer water to give you that same bubbly feeling, without the caffeine, added sugar or artificial sweetener that's in most soda pop. Have plain seltzer with some lemon and lime wedges for your own version of a lemon-lime pop. Make a juice spritzer by pouring a very small amount of 100% juice (just for flavor) in the bottom of a glass and filling the glass up the rest of the way with seltzer. Voila! You've made a great beverage choice.

Chapter 6

I don't have the time
or the money for exercise!

A gym is not the only place you can get exercise, by any means. For everyone, some exercise is better than not getting any at all. So walk! Walking is the best way to accomplish what you need to do and exercise at the same time. Moderate-intensity exercise like walking is safe for nearly everyone to do.[14] If you have a chronic condition such as diabetes, arthritis, or heart disease, work with your doctor on which exercises are right for you. For most of us, you can add walking and other exercises to things you already do as part of your daily routine. If you're in a walkable community and you need to run an errand down the street, walk there! If you're not too sure about this, remember that most of us need to make time for exercise. Think about exercising like any other appointment or meeting you might have. Write it into your day planner or agenda. Make a schedule of what you'd like to do for exercise and post it somewhere you will see it every day, as an extra reminder.

Hope's Handy Hint: Moving around more often throughout the day (like the ideas listed below) may help move those air bubbles through your gut swiftly so you have under-the-radar cute little toots instead of noisy, juicy ones or the notorious SBD (silent but deadly). An incentive for exercise, perhaps?

- At a strip mall park in a central location and walk from store to car to store, without moving the car
- Walk on your lunch break
- Take a lap around the grocery store or mall before you start to do your shopping
- Carry grocery bags in one at a time, instead of trying to do it all at once

[14] Centers for Disease Control and Prevention. (2008). *Physical activity for everyone: Physical activity and health.* Retrieved August 26, 2009 from http://www.cdc.gov/physicalactivity/everyone/health/index.html.

- Walk in place or around the room when on the phone
- Walk around the house during TV commercial breaks
- Disengage the self-propelling feature of your lawn mower so you're actually pushing it
- Put a mini bike or mini stepper under your desk at work and use it while doing computer work
- Sit on a stability disk at work or on an exercise ball
- Use a restroom on another floor when you're at work
- Find a fun exercise video you can do at home or with a workout buddy (check out local libraries)
- Take the stairs instead of the elevator
- Dance to fun music for 5 minutes each day when you're getting ready for work or school
- Do push-ups for 5 minutes when you wake up; stretch for 5 minutes before you go to bed
- Take a walk with your family after dinner instead of watching TV
- Curl water bottles, soup cans, or dumbbells while watching TV

Chapter 7

Tell me what I need to eat, and when to eat it!

You might not want to hear any more about "why" you need to eat this or that or "what" it helps you with. You want an exact diet to follow for a few weeks (or as long as you can stand it) so you can lose weight and get it over with. I bet you'd like to have someone like me do your food shopping and prepare all your meals and snacks, so you just have to show up. Unfortunately, that's not the real world and is not actually going to help you. **A "diet" is something that you do short-term. What you need to do is to make lifestyle changes, so you actually improve or maintain your health and body weight**. Use this information to help you stay healthy for the long-term. You need to learn **ON YOUR OWN** how to come up with a healthful eating plan (notice it's not a DIET) that works for you. I want to help you to reach that goal. Use this template to help you keep your body fueled evenly throughout the day and to meet all the different food group goals.

Hope's Handy Hint: Do not skip meals. Notice that this template involves eating 5 times a day. **Snacks are not taboo** – in fact, snacks will become your best friend (the third wheel with you and those grocery circulars). That's because you don't want to go too long between times that you eat. When you wait too long to eat not only do you get crabby, you probably will eat more at the next meal and maybe overeat. Also, eating consistently throughout the day may help you to feel better and to make wiser food choices, since you're not going through those crabby I-need-something-to-eat-now-or-I'll-hurt-someone phases.

The general pattern to follow looks like this, for the calorie levels listed.

	1600 calories	1800 calories	2000 calories	2200 calories	2400 calories
Breakfast	2 oz grain ½ cup milk ¾ cup fruit ½ oz protein	2 oz grain ½ cup milk 1 cup fruit ½ oz protein	2 oz grain ½ cup milk 1 ¼ cups fruit 1 oz protein	2 ½ oz grain ¾ cup milk 1 ½ cup fruit 1 oz protein	2 ½ oz grain ¾ cup milk 1 ½ cup fruit 1 oz protein
Snack*	¾ cup milk ½ cup fruit	¾ cup milk ½ cup fruit	¾ cup milk ½ cup fruit	¾ cup milk ½ cup fruit	¾ cup milk ½ cup fruit
Lunch	¾ cup milk 1 ½ oz protein 1 ½ oz grain ½ cup vegetables with 1 tsp fat	¾ cup milk 1 ½ oz protein 1 ½ oz grain ¾ cup vegetables with 1 tsp fat	¾ cup milk 1 ½ oz protein 1 ½ oz grain ¾ cup vegetables with 1 tsp fat	¾ cup milk 2 ½ oz protein 1 ½ oz grain ¾ cup vegetables with 1 tsp fat	¾ cup milk 2 ½ oz protein 2 ½ oz grain ¾ cup vegetables with 1 tsp fat
Snack	¼ cup milk ½ oz grain ½ cup vegetables	¼ cup milk ½ oz grain ¾ cup vegetables	¼ cup milk ½ oz grain ¾ cup vegetables	¼ cup milk 1 ½ oz grain ¾ cup vegetables	¼ cup milk 1 ½ oz grain ¾ cup vegetables
Dinner	¾ cup milk 3 oz protein 1 oz grain 1 cup vegetables with 2 tsp fat	¾ cup milk 3 oz protein 1 ½ oz grain 1 cup vegetables with 2 tsp fat	¾ cup milk 3 oz protein 1 ½ oz grain 1 cup vegetables with 2 tsp fat	¾ cup milk 3 oz protein 1 ½ oz grain 1 ½ cups vegetables with 2 tsp fat	¾ cup milk 3 oz protein 1 ½ oz grain 1 ½ cups vegetables with 2 tsp fat
Dessert	1 dark chocolate candy bar (1.45 oz size)	1 dark chocolate candy bar (2 oz size)	1 dark chocolate candy bar (2 oz size)	1 dark chocolate candy bar (2.25 oz size)	1 dark chocolate candy bar (3 oz size)

Based on: U.S. Department of Agriculture, Center for Nutrition Policy and Promotion. (April 2005). *MyPyramid: Food intake patterns.*
* This snack could also be used after dinner, if you prefer to eat something after dinner and before bed.

At this point you might be wondering about ounces of grain and protein. Although it's more of that unwanted nutrition education, a little background information will help you immensely. The food pyramid comes from the *Dietary Guidelines for Americans*, which is published by the U.S. government every 5 years. The newest food pyramid, called MyPyramid, is internet-based and was developed from the 2005 *Dietary Guidelines for Americans*. The following information on portion sizes is from www.mypyramid.gov, the website for the new food pyramid.

What counts as an ounce of grain?

- 1 slice of bread (slightly smaller than a CD)
- 1 cup of cold cereal (size of your fist, or a tennis ball)
- ½ cup of cooked rice, cooked pasta, or cooked cereal (size of ½ a tennis ball, or a cupcake wrapper)
- 1 "mini" bagel (size of a hockey puck)
- ½ English muffin
- 5 whole wheat crackers
- 1-4 ½" pancake (size of a CD)
- 3 cups popcorn
- 1 packet plain instant oatmeal
- 1 – 6" tortilla (slightly bigger than a CD)

What counts as an ounce equivalent of protein?

- 1 egg = 1 oz
- 1 Tbsp peanut butter = 1 oz (1/2 a ping-pong ball)
- ¼ c (about 2 oz) tofu = 1 oz
- 2 Tbsp hummus = 1 oz
- 1 small steak = 3 ½ - 4 oz (a deck of playing cards)
- 1 small lean hamburger = 2-3 oz
- 1 salmon steak = 4-6 oz (a computer mouse)
- 1 can tuna, drained = 3-4 oz
- 24 almonds, 48 pistachios, 14 walnut halves = 2 oz
- 1 cup split pea soup, lentil soup, or bean soup = 2 oz
- 1 soy burger or bean patty = 2 oz

What counts as 1 cup of fruit?

- ½ large apple, or 1 small apple (the size of a baseball)
- 1 large banana
- 1 large peach, or 2 halves canned
- 8 large strawberries

- 32 seedless grapes
- 1 medium grapefruit (4" diameter)
- 1 medium pear
- 3 medium or 2 large plums
- 1 small watermelon wedge

- 1 large orange
- ½ cup dried fruit (a cupcake wrapper)

What counts as 1 cup of vegetables?

In general, 1 cup of raw or cooked vegetables or vegetable juice or 2 cups of raw leafy greens can be considered as 1 cup. 1 cup is about the size of a fist. Other vegetables equaling 1 cup:

- 2 medium carrots, or 12 baby carrots
- 1 large baked sweet potato
- About 8 oz tofu (1 cup ½" cubes)
- 1 medium boiled or baked white potato

- 2 large stalks of celery
- 1 large ear of corn
- 1 large pepper
- 1 large raw whole tomato (3")

What counts as a serving of milk?

- 1 cup of milk or yogurt
- 8 oz container of yogurt (6 oz container = ¾ cup, 4 oz snack size = ½ cup)
- 1 ½ oz hard Cheese (cheddar, Mozzarella, Swiss, parmesan) (the size of your thumb)

- 1/3 cup shredded cheese
- 2 oz processed cheese (1 slice of American cheese = 1/3 cup; 3 slices = 2oz = 1 serving)
- 2 cups cottage cheese (½ cup, about a cupcake wrapper = ¼ cup milk)

- 1 cup pudding made with milk
- 1 cup frozen yogurt

Earlier we discussed how many calories you should eat based on your gender, age, and exercise level. To lose 1 pound per week, you need to take in 500 fewer calories per day than what's recommended. To lose ½ a pound per week, take in 250 fewer calories per day. Reverse this to gain weight – add 250 calories per day to gain ½ a pound per week, 500 calories a day to gain 1 pound per week. **Do not consume fewer than 1600 calories per day without talking to your doctor**. By eating fewer than 1600 calories per day, you might not get enough of the vitamins, minerals, and other nutrients you need. And a multivitamin cannot make up for poor or inadequate eating habits.

Hope's Handy Hint: Here's an example of how to adjust your calorie level to lose weight.

A 27 year old woman is walking briskly for 45 minutes a day, 6 days of the week. For this amount of exercise she needs to eat 2000 calories per day. This woman would like to lose weight. To lose about ½ a pound per week, she needs 1800 calories per day (instead of 2000). If she wants to increase the amount of weight she's losing each week, she could stick with 1800 calories but increase the amount of time she's walking to 60 minutes per day.

Now, put together how many calories per day you need, with the calorie level you'll need if you want to lose/gain/maintain your weight, and the meal pattern for that calorie level.

The following is a 1-day sample menu for different calorie levels. This will help you see how to apply that general pattern to real-world eating. You'll notice that each menu plan is the same, with just a few slight variations to adjust the amount of calories. One reason for this is so you can see easily how to adjust from one calorie level to another. A second reason is so that everyone in your house can eat basically the same way. Meals can be shared, foods can all be prepared at one time, and you can enjoy life a little more. No one wants to be a short-order cook at home. Use this as an example for you to come up with your own healthful eating plans. Enjoy!

1-Day Menu Plan for 1600 Calories

Breakfast	1 slice raisin bread with ½ tbsp peanut butter ¾ cup Cheerios with ½ cup skim milk ½ medium peach and ½ cup blueberries
Snack	6 oz low fat yogurt and 16 cherries
Lunch	1 large slice of bread (cut in half) with 2 cooked egg whites (lettuce & tomato optional) ¾ cup of milk ½ cup cooked snow peas with 1 tsp whipped butter
Snack	½ cup low fat cottage cheese with 6 baby carrots and 3 reduced-fat triscuits
Dinner	¾ cup skim milk ½ cup cooked brown rice with 1 tsp whipped butter ½ cup cooked cauliflower and ½ cup cooked broccoli, with 1 tsp whipped butter 1 medium baked/grilled chicken breast (without skin, 3 oz meat) with a small amount of barbeque sauce
Dessert	1 dark chocolate candy bar (1.45 oz size)
Provides: 1579 calories, 95 grams protein, 213 grams carbohydrate, 24 grams fiber, 45 grams fat (19.7 grams sat. fat, 16 grams mono. Fat, 6 grams poly. Fat), 112 mg cholesterol, 1220 mg calcium, 2535 mg sodium	

1-Day Menu Plan for 1800 calories

Breakfast	1 slice raisin bread with ½ tbsp peanut butter 1 cup Cheerios with ½ cup skim milk ½ medium peach and ½ cup blueberries
Snack	6 oz low fat yogurt and 16 cherries
Lunch	1 large slice of bread (cut in half) with 2 cooked egg whites (lettuce & tomato optional) ¾ cup of milk ¾ cup cooked snow peas with 1 tsp whipped butter
Snack	½ cup low fat cottage cheese with 8 baby carrots and 3 reduced-fat triscuits
Dinner	1 cup skim milk ¾ cup cooked brown rice with 1 tsp whipped butter ½ cup cooked cauliflower and ½ cup cooked broccoli, with 1 tsp whipped butter 1 medium baked/grilled chicken breast (without skin, 3 oz meat) with a small amount of barbeque sauce
Dessert	1 dark chocolate bar (2.2 oz)
Provides: 1818 calories, 101 grams protein, 249 grams carbohydrate, 28 grams fiber, 54 grams fat (24 grams sat. fat, 19 grams mono. Fat, 7 grams poly. Fat), 113 mg cholesterol, 1353 mg calcium, 2743 mg sodium	

1-Day Menu Plan for 2000 calories

Breakfast	1 slice raisin bread with 1 tbsp peanut butter 1 cup Cheerios with 1/2 cup skim milk 1 medium peach and ¾ cup blueberries
Snack	6 oz low fat yogurt and 16 cherries
Lunch	2 large slices of bread with 2 cooked egg whites (lettuce & tomato optional) ¾ cup of milk ¾ cup cooked snow peas with 1 tsp whipped butter
Snack	½ cup low fat cottage cheese with 8 baby carrots and 3 reduced-fat triscuits
Dinner	¾ cup skim milk ¾ cup cooked brown rice with 1 tsp whipped butter ½ cup cooked cauliflower and ½ cup cooked broccoli, with 1 tsp whipped butter 1 medium baked/grilled chicken breast (without skin, 3 oz meat) with a small amount of barbeque sauce
Dessert	2 small dark chocolate bars (1.45 oz each)
Provides: 2059 calories, 104 grams protein, 284 grams carbohydrate, 33 grams fiber, 67 grams fat (29.4 grams sat. fat, 24 grams mono. Fat, 9 grams poly. Fat), 112 mg cholesterol, 1307.5 mg calcium, 2863 mg sodium	

1-Day Menu Plan for 2200 calories

Breakfast	1 slice raisin bread with 1 tbsp peanut butter 1 ½ cup Cheerios with ¾ cup skim milk ½ medium peach and 1 cup blueberries
Snack	6 oz low fat yogurt and 16 cherries
Lunch	2 large slices of bread with 2 cooked egg whites (lettuce & tomato optional) ¾ cup of milk ¾ cup cooked snow peas with 1 tsp whipped butter 11 whole almonds
Snack	½ cup low fat cottage cheese with 8 baby carrots and 7 reduced-fat triscuits
Dinner	¾ cup skim milk ¾ cup cooked brown rice with 1 tsp whipped butter ¾ cup cooked cauliflower and ¾ cup cooked broccoli, with 1 tsp whipped butter 1 medium baked/grilled chicken breast (without skin, 3 oz meat) with a small amount of barbeque sauce
Snack	2 oz dark chocolate bar
Provides: 2178 calories, 114 grams protein, 298 grams carbohydrate, 39 grams fiber, 69 grams fat (25 grams sat. fat, 28 grams mono. Fat, 12 grams poly. Fat), 113 mg cholesterol, 1493.5 mg calcium, 3371 mg sodium	

1-Day Menu Plan for 2400 calories

Breakfast	1 slice raisin bread with 1 tbsp peanut butter 1 ½ cup Cheerios with ¾ cup skim milk ½ medium peach and 1 cup blueberries
Snack	6 oz low fat yogurt and 16 cherries
Lunch	2 large slices of bread with 2 cooked egg whites (lettuce & tomato optional) ¾ cup of milk ¾ cup cooked snow peas with 1 tsp whipped butter 11 whole almonds
Snack	½ cup low fat cottage cheese with 8 baby carrots and 9 reduced-fat triscuits
Dinner	¾ cup skim milk 1 cup cooked brown rice with 1 tsp whipped butter ¾ cup cooked cauliflower and ¾ cup cooked broccoli, with 1 tsp whipped butter 1 medium baked/grilled chicken breast (without skin, 3 oz meat) with a small amount of barbeque sauce
Dessert	2 small dark chocolate bars (1.45 oz each)
Provides: 2409 calories, 117 grams protein, 333 grams carbohydrate, 42 grams fiber, 80 grams fat (31 grams sat. fat, 31 grams mono. Fat, 12 grams poly. Fat), 113 mg cholesterol, 1508.2 mg calcium, 3409 mg sodium	

All menus were analyzed for nutritional content using MyPyramid Tracker, available free at http://www.mypyramidtracker.gov/.

Chapter 8

Healthful Recipes Your Family Will Love!

Wait! Where are the recipes? They seem to have fallen out of the book...

GOTCHA! Actually, there are no recipes in this book. I have no idea what your favorite recipes are or what types of meals your family enjoys. I'm not going to impose some totally new and different recipes on you that have ingredients with names you might not be able to pronounce. What I am going to do, however, is to help you to **START with the recipes you already have and know how to make**. There's always room for improvement!

Like we talked about in chapter 3, **make over some of your typical meals and recipes in order to make them more healthful**. Simple modifications are usually the best way to eat better and to avoid a mutiny in your home.

A few examples to try:

- Make oven-fried chicken instead of regular (skillet-cooked) fried chicken
- Use oatmeal for breadcrumbs
- Add more beans and less meat to chili and meatloaf
- Make half the flour in baked goods whole wheat
- Use applesauce for ½ the oil in a recipe
- Make pancakes with low fat yogurt instead of with oil and eggs
- Use egg white or egg substitute in omelets and baked goods
- Add more veggies and less meat on a pizza, and have a salad along with the pizza
- Put fat-free plain yogurt on a baked potato instead of sour cream
- Spread a light coat of natural PB on toast instead of butter
- Use nonstick cooking spray to grease pans instead of shortening, butter, or lard

This is just a small sample of what you can do! As you try some of these ideas you'll start to come up with lots of other ways to incorporate what you've learned here into your everyday cooking. It takes a little trial-and-error, so see what works best for you and anyone else for whom you're preparing foods.

Chapter 9

Get moving!

Hope's Handy Hint: Remember that some exercise is better than no exercise at all, so don't be discouraged if you have some "on" weeks and some "off" weeks. Do what you can with what you've got.

In 2008 the U.S. government released the very first *Physical Activity Guidelines for Americans*. This is exactly what it sounds like – a guide to type, time, and intensity of exercise we need.

Group:	Time:	Intensity:	Special Notes:
Kids and Teenagers (age 6-17)	At least 60 minutes of exercise each day	Moderate or vigorous-intensity	Vigorous intensity activity at least 3 days a week; muscle-strengthening activity at least 3 days a week
Kids and Teenagers With Disabilities	Follow guidelines for kids and teenagers		Work with healthcare provider to identify appropriate activities to meet guidelines; Be as physically active as possible; avoid inactivity
Adults (age 18 – 64)	At least: • 2 hours and 30 minutes a week OR • 1 hour and 15 minutes (75 minutes) OR • A combination of both	• Moderate-intensity • Vigorous-intensity • Moderate and vigorous-intensity	At least 10 minutes of exercise at a time; do muscle-strengthening activities at least 2 days a week.
Adults with Disabilities	Follow adult guidelines		Be as physically active as possible; avoid inactivity

Group:	Time:	Intensity:	Special Notes:
Older Adults (age 65 and older)	Follow adult guidelines		Be as physically active as abilities allow; avoid inactivity; do exercises that maintain or improve balance if at risk of falling
Pregnant and New Moms	At least 2 hours and 30 minutes a week	Moderate - intensity	Spread activity throughout the week; if already doing vigorous-intensity aerobic activity can continue activity, provided condition remains unchanged and have discussed activity level with health care provider

Source: U.S. Department of Health and Human Services. (2008). At-a-glance: A fact sheet for professionals. *2008 Physical Activity Guidelines for Americans.* Retrieved August 24, 2009 from http://www.health.gov/paguidelines/factsheetprof.aspx.

You might be asking yourself what the heck moderate or vigorous-intensity exercise means. The **"talk test"**[15] is a good way to know how intensely you are exercising. If you're too winded to sing while you're exercising but you can still **carry on a conversation**, you're doing **moderate-intensity** exercise. If you're **too winded to sing or even to talk**, you're doing **vigorous-intensity** exercise.

General activities considered to be **moderate-intensity** include[15]:

- Brisk walking indoors or outdoors ($\geq$ 3 miles per hour)
- Water aerobics
- Bicycling indoors or outdoors (slower than 10 miles per hour)
- Doubles tennis
- General Gardening

General activities considered to be **vigorous-intensity** include[15]:

- Race walking, jogging, or running indoors or outdoors
- Swimming laps
- Singles tennis
- Jumping rope
- Aerobic dancing
- Continuous digging or hoeing in a garden/yard
- Hiking uphill or with a heavy pack

Remember that being "fit" isn't just being able to lift really heavy boxes, running the fastest or having the best aim. Many people can go to the gym every day without actually being fit. Physical fitness[16] is a combination of many different factors. To be fit, you need to have:

- Cardio respiratory endurance (aerobic or lung power)
- Muscle endurance (your muscles' "staying power")
- Muscle strength (ability to exert force)
- Muscle power (how efficiently your muscles can contract)
- Flexibility (the range of motion possible at a joint)
- Balance
- Speed of movement
- Reaction time

---

[15] Centers for Disease Control and Prevention. (2009). *Physical activity for everyone: Measuring physical activity intensity.* Retrieved September 29, 2009 from http://www.cdc.gov/physicalactivity/everyone/measuring/index.html.
[16] Centers for Disease Control and Prevention. (2008). *Physical activity for everyone: Glossary of terms.* Retrieved August 17, 2009 from http://www.cdc.gov/physicalactivity/everyone/glossary/index.html.

- Body composition (how much of your body is fat and how much is muscle)

The 2008 Physical *Activity Guidelines* sound much more confusing than they actually are. It helps to see the recommendations broken down into a week of exercise. There are many different ways and different combinations to get the exercise that's recommended.

To get the lowest amount of exercise that's recommended, try:

Monday	Tuesday	Wednesday	Thursday	Friday	Total
30 minute walk OR 15 minute walk in AM + 15 minute walk in PM	30 minute walk + Strength Training	30 minute walk OR 15 minute walk in AM + 15 minute walk in PM	30 minute walk + Strength Training	30 minute walk OR 15 minute walk in AM + 15 minute walk in PM	150 minutes moderate-intensity exercise + 2 days strength training

Or:

Monday	Tuesday	Wednesday	Thursday	Friday	Total
25 minute jog	Strength Training	25 minute jog	Strength Training	25 minute jog	75 minutes vigorous-intensity exercise + 2 days strength training

Or a combination of moderate- and vigorous-intensity exercises:

Monday	Tuesday	Wednesday	Thursday	Friday	Total
30 minutes water aerobics	Yoga & 15 minute walk	30 minute jog	Yoga & 15 minute walk	30 minute walk	90 minutes moderate-intensity exercise + 30 minutes vigorous intensity exercise + 2 days strength training

Remember that these are examples of the minimum amount of exercise recommended. By increasing to 5 hours a week of moderate-intensity exercise, 2 ½ hours a week of vigorous-intensity exercise, or a combination of both, you'll get greater health benefits. To lose weight, you may need to increase your exercise to 60 minutes a day; to keep the weight off once you've lost it, you may need to increase your exercise to 60 to 90 minutes a day.[17]

Once you've conquered 30 minutes of exercise, 5 days a week, gradually increase your exercise to 1 hour on most days of the week. For example, each week for 3 weeks increase your exercise by 10 minutes a day. You'll feel a huge sense of accomplishment when you've made it to a full hour of exercise!

---

[17] U.S. Department of Health and Human Services. (2005). Chapter 3: Weight management. *Dietary Guidelines for Americans, 2005*: Retrieved August 31, 2009 from http://www.health.gov/dietaryguidelines/dga2005/document/html/chapter3.htm.

To get the amount of exercise needed for weight loss and weight maintenance, try:

Monday	Tuesday	Wednesday	Thursday	Friday	Saturday	Sunday	Total
30 minute walk in AM +15 minute walk at lunch + 15 minute walk in PM	15 minute walk in AM and Strength Training +15 minute walk at lunch + 30 minute walk in PM	30 minute walk in AM +15 minute walk at lunch + 15 minute walk in PM	15 minute walk in AM and Strength Training +15 minute walk at lunch + 30 minute walk in PM	30 minute walk in AM +15 minute walk at lunch + 15 minute walk in PM	30 minutes Mowing grass (push mower) + 30 minutes vacuuming	REST	6 hours moderate-intensity exercise + 2 days strength training

Or:

Monday	Tuesday	Wednesday	Thursday	Friday	Saturday	Sunday	Total
30 minute jog	Strength Training + 15 minute jog	30 minute jog	Strength Training + 15 minute jog	30 minute jog	30 minute jog	REST	150 minutes vigorous-intensity exercise + 2 days strength training

Or a combination of moderate- and vigorous-intensity exercises:

Monday	Tuesday	Wednesday	Thursday	Friday	Saturday	Sunday	Total
30 minutes water aerobics + 30 minute walk	Yoga & 30 minute walk OR Yoga + 15 minute walk at lunch + 15 minute walk in evening	30 minute jog	Yoga & 30 minute walk OR Yoga + 15 minute walk at lunch + 15 minute walk in evening	60 minute walk OR 20 minute walk in AM + 20 minute walk at lunch + 20 minute walk in evening	30 minute jog	REST	180 minutes moderate-intensity exercise + 60 minutes vigorous intensity exercise + 2 days strength training

Conclusion

You probably have figured it out by now, but the purpose of this book is **_not_** essentially to help you lose weight. It's to help you think about how you're living now and the changes you may need to make in order to live a healthy life. When your life is healthy, you'll be at a healthy body weight. The best "diet" is to have a healthy lifestyle that you can keep up with your entire life. To keep your body healthy and to be at a healthy weight, you need to make healthful food choices, have sensible portions, and put exercise into your everyday routine. This helps you as an individual, but it also helps everyone around you, our healthcare system, our country, and the world in general.

A rhyme for you as we bid adieu:

> Fiber is a magical fuel
> Fruits & veggies & whole grains rule!
> Make healthful choices & watch portion sizes,
> A healthy weight will be one of your prizes!
> Exercise, exercise everyday
> Watch the pounds melt away!
> Make small changes – don't go crazy
> But keep up with it and don't be lazy.
> Take care of your body and it'll take care of you
> Our wish for world peace might then come true!

Best of luck,

Dietitian Hope

Index